PETER'S FOOT

RSD

Calmare® Scrambler Therapy

Experienced

by

Peter Hinninger

Words & Photos

by

Judy Alberta

This book

is dedicated

to the loved ones

in our lives.

Copyright © 2017 Peter Hinninger & Judy Alberta

All rights reserved.

ISBN: 13:978-1974217205

You are reading this book because you or someone you love is suffering with chronic, burning, unrelenting pain and has been diagnosed with RSD or CRPS.

You are searching for information and relief from this cruel, debilitating, burning pain.

Peter and I discovered Calmare® Therapy..

Knowing. first hand, what it is like to endure RSD we are eager to share with you what we discovered and experienced in July 2017 for two weeks of Calmare® Therapy.

The Calmare® Therapy Treatment was and continues to be successful in vanquishing Peter's burning RSD pain.

We are hopeful that you will find our day by day account of the Calmare® Treatment informative, helpful and will also soon be happily pain free.

                Sincerely,

                Judy and Peter

Seventeen years ago, September 11, 2000, a car accident. Peter was hit from behind by a tractor trailer. The accident crushed his car and his right foot and split open his pelvis. Twenty-eight bones were broken. The doctors at Jersey Shore Medical did an incredible job of putting him back together. He defied the odds by relearning to walk a year after the accident.

Peter's bones and skin healed, but his nerves did not. For seventeen years he has suffered severe, chronic, and continuous, pain, more specifically the sensation of burning oil being poured on his right foot. The condition is called Reflex Sympathetic Dystrophy(RSD).

Peter has consulted with many specialists and tried a multitude of treatments for RSD including spinal blocks, ganglion blocks, spinal cord stimulator, Lyrica®, Morphine, and Fentanyl. All of which resulted in minimal relief from the constant burning pain in both feet and sometimes up both legs. Three to five or sometimes more Oxycodone per day helped alleviate some of the pain, but the Oxycodone was causing side effects.

The disease was getting progressively worse. Peter was taking more and more Oxycodone. Sometimes he would not eat for days. His stomach was often upset and he was losing weight rapidly. Little hope was left for any relief from the burning pain that would begin in his right foot and travel to the sympathetic left foot, often migrating to include the entire right leg and part of his pelvis.

When we, quite by chance, came across the Calmare® Treatment, it was viewed with skepticism but then a thin shred of hope pushed to the surface. Arrangements were made to begin treatment.

Dr. Michael Cooney

RUTHERFORD ALLIED MEDICAL GROUP

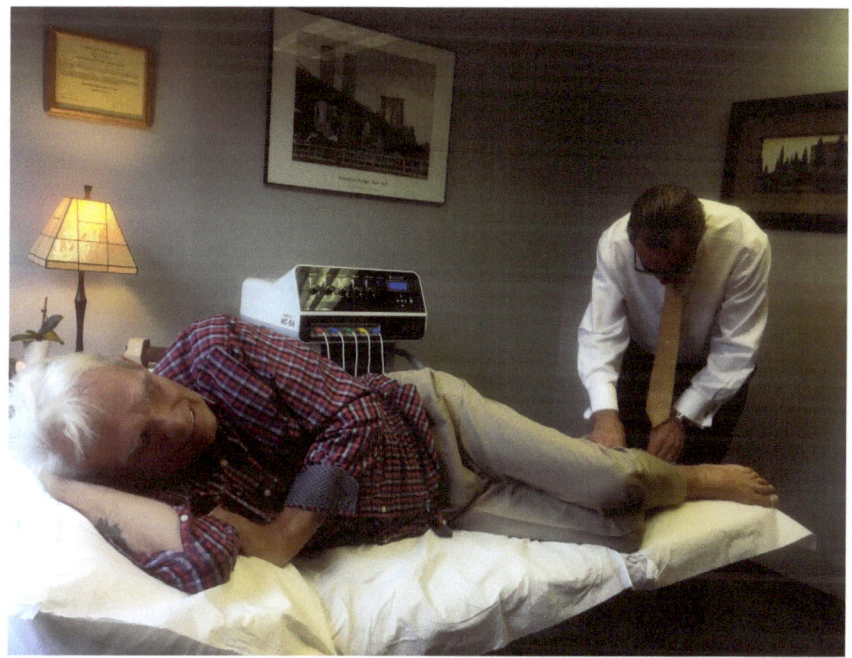

Peter arrives at Dr. Cooney's Rutherford Allied Medical Group office in Rutherford New Jersey with a persistent level eight pain in his right foot. He has difficulty standing because his right foot, in addition to the burning pain, feels the size of a football.

Peter's mind is so preoccupied coping with the pain he is unable to fill in the information for the payment check. He scratches his signature and I fill in the necessary check information.

The cost for 10 treatments is $3,000

Dr. Cooney asks Peter several questions about his pain, location and history. Treatment begins with five sets of electrode pairs affixed to Peter's back and foot.

Each set connects to the Calmare® Machine.

Dr. Cooney adjusts the current on each line separately.

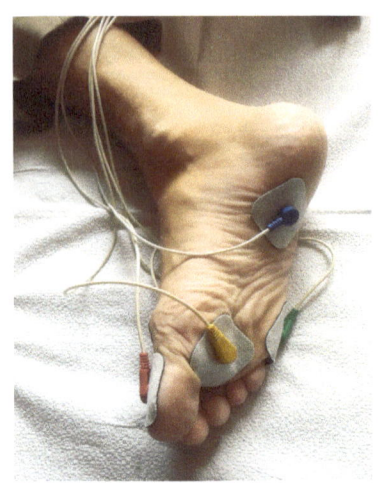

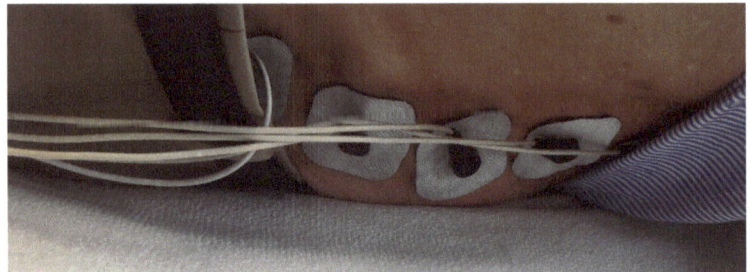

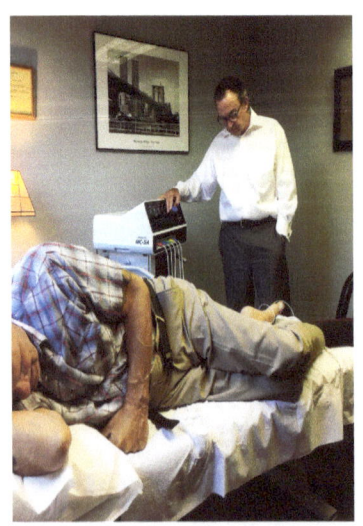

When Peter feels the current for each line he lets Dr. Cooney know and that is where the level stays for the 35 minutes of treatment. The current is never at a painful level. Peter remarks, "It feels good, like a massage".

The pain is at level 2 at the end of the 35 minutes of treatment!

How Calmare® Scrambler Therapy Work?

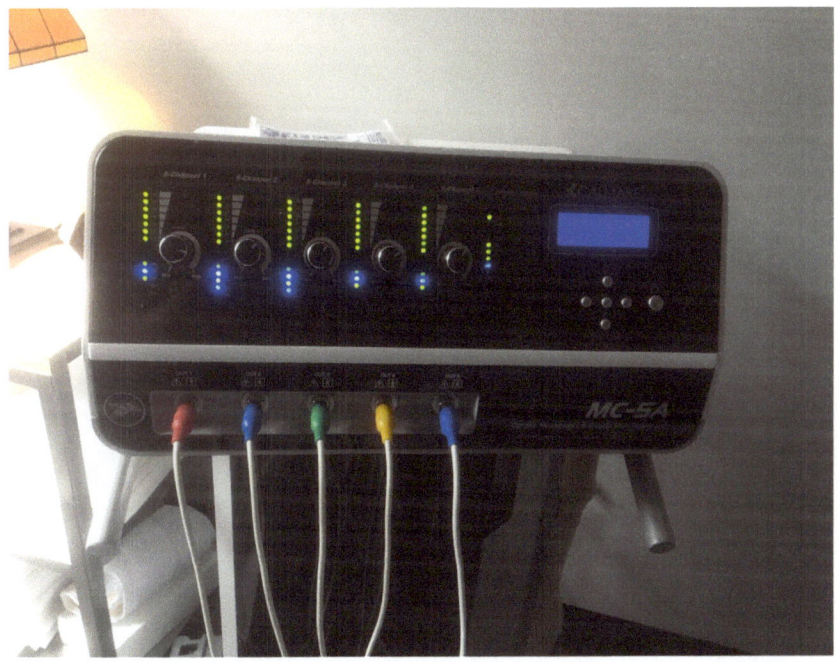

This is information from the Calmare® web site. "The Calmare® Therapy machine uses a biophysical (using physical methods) rather than a biochemical (drugs) approach. The device relieves pain directly at the pain site through small electrodes producing a no-pain message which is transmitted directly to the nerve for about 35 minutes using 16 distinct algorithms."

The lights on the machine jump up and down as the machine changes the electrical impulses to each line. Peter can feel the impulse shifts in his back, legs, right foot and in his left sympathetic foot.

The Treatments are Monday to Friday for a Two-week Period.

Peter and I live about two hours from Rutherford. We planned to commute. That idea, we immediately realized, was not realistic.

After the first treatment Peter was very tired. His need for sleep and the stress of traffic would make traveling impossible and we felt this would not aid the treatment process.

We booked the Residence Marriott for two weeks and took advantage of the discount offered by The Rutherford Allied Medical Group.

Marriott Residence Inn

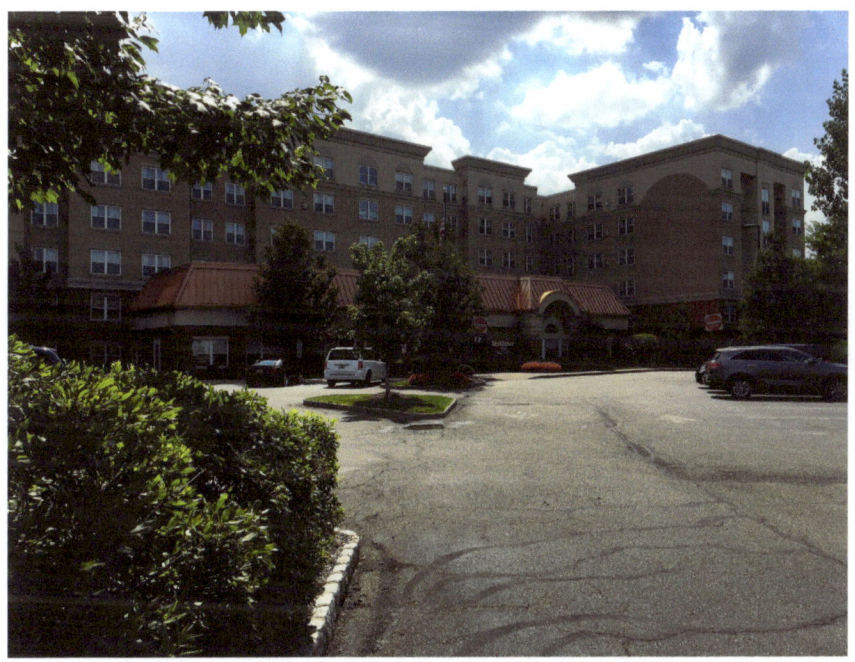

The Marriott Residence Inn is a short distance from Dr. Cooney's office. The Inn offers a beautiful and varied complimentary buffet breakfast each morning. Scrambled eggs, sausage, fresh fruit, yogurt, cereal, waffles, orange juice, coffee and tea were the choices.

It was a treat to wake up and have breakfast waiting for us.

On Monday, Tuesday and Wednesday a light dinner was available.

Our room has a comfortable king size bed in a separate area. There is also a sofa and chair in a living space, a kitchen, a dining table, and a desk. The large flat screen television swiveled so it could be seen from all areas.

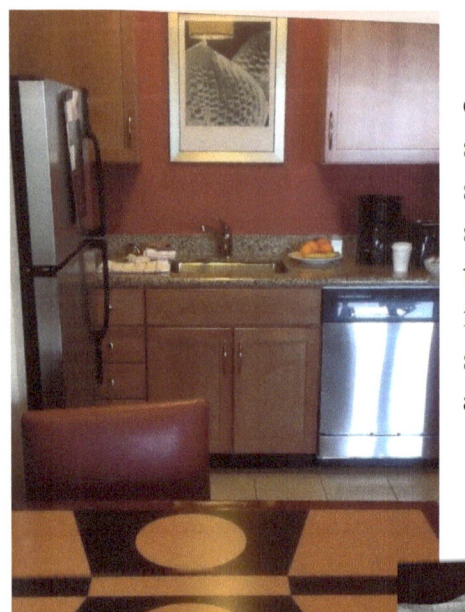

Sleepiness is a definite side effect of the treatment. Going out to eat was beyond Peter's energy level and ability to stay awake. The small kitchen in the room was well used and appreciated. We ate lunch and dinner in the room every night untill Wednesday of the second week of treatment.

The following is a copy of the text messages sent to family every day during the first week of the Calmare® treatment.

WEEK ONE

July 10, 2017, Monday, Week 1, Treatment 1:

Arrive at office with a level 8 pain. After treatment the pain is at a level 2. This reduction in pain lasted for a wonderful 6 hours.

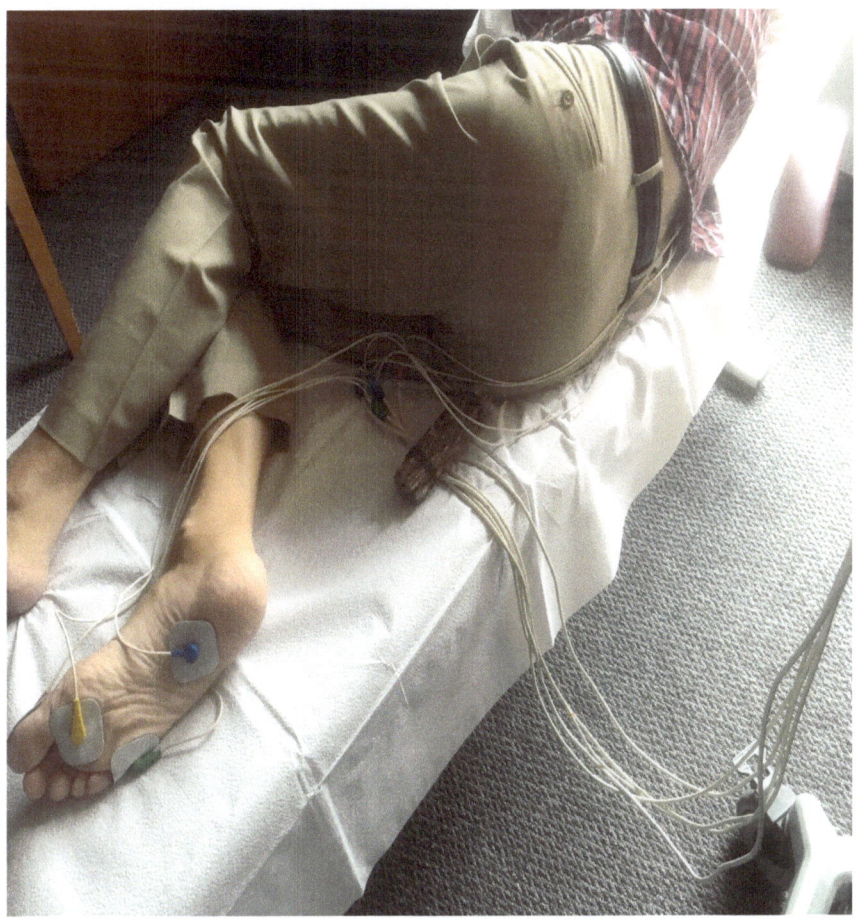

Tuesday, Week 1, Treatment 2:

Peter arrived for treatment today in full pain choosing NOT to take a pain pill. By the time the 35-minute treatment was complete the burning and pain were minimal. The doctor is very pleased that the pain took about 6+ hours to return. (he anticipated 4hrs.) Six is a very good indicator of success. He anticipates it will be even longer with today's treatment. Other than sleepiness (which is a side effect of the treatment) Peter is very optimistic. Pain is gone!

Wednesday, Week 1, Treatment 3:

Good Morning. This is so incredible! No, Nada, Zip, Zero pain since after yesterday's treatment! An amazing 19 hours and counting! Peter spent most of the night looking at his foot in disbelief and fearfully waiting for the pain to rear it's ugly head. Peter remains pain free this morning. This is amazing and after only 2 treatments! I had to tell Peter he probably shouldn't dance on the tables at breakfast!

Peter continues to enjoy a pain free, non burning foot. He is extremely tired and sleeps continuously, about 20 hours a day. Dr. Cooney said that no pain for an extended period of time on a second visit is excellent! The sleeping is expected and a side effect of the brain reprogramming itself. I wake Peter for meals and he is eating a good amount of food. His appetite is returning. His stomach is a little upset now but a big glass of milk is making him feel better. Experiencing no pain is new and unfamiliar to his body along with a reduction in pain pills needed for pain. He plans to wean himself with a half a pill for a while to adjust.

Wed. night: Peter slept through the night without waking. This is the first time he can remember not waking to burning pain in the middle of the night. Eating well. Feeling "normal'. 😊.

Thursday, Week 1, Treatment 4:

Dr. Cooney is very pleased with Peter's progress. He said usually people who come in with a level 8 pain after the first week of treatment drop to a level 4. Then after the second week continue dropping to perhaps a level 2. Peter dropped to a 0 after his second visit. This is an amazing result and he predicts an indicator of an extremely good pattern.

Friday, Week 1, Treatment 5:

In addition to being pain free there is a return of feeling in Peter's big toe and the side of his right foot. Peter's right foot has been numb for years. Where his foot had a bluish tinge now appears normal in color. The feeling of a thick skin on foot, as Peter calls it "Elephant Skin" is less. Extreme sleepiness is still a side effect but, when Peter is awake he is grinning from ear to ear!

Treatment is today at 11 in the morning.

We decided to return home for the weekend.

We kept the room. Checking out on Friday and checking back in on Monday cost the same because the discount would not be in effect. This makes it easy to return on Monday morning. We left some clothes in the closet and food in the fridge. On a day like today, overcast, wet and drizzling Peter's pain level and aches would be at their worst. Today this wet, humid, cloudy day he is driving and pain free. Peter is very happy and very excited to be heading home.

No treatment untill 2:00 on Monday is a scary thought. What will happen? Dr. Cooney said the pain could remain a level 0 or it could return. If the pain does return do not be surprised or disheartened. If it does it will most likely be at a lesser degree.

Saturday

Peter woke at 2:00PM from a nap with a level 4 pain with a burning sensation on top and bottom of right foot. To a lesser extent on the left. Unpleasant but not excruciating. Took one pain pill at 2:10. At 2:35 there was 0 pain.

Prior to treatment the pain would have been reduced by the pill. Peter states. "Now I'm asymptomatic rather than in the past I would get a slight relief from the pain but not complete relief from the pain." The pain pill would have lasted about three hours, whereas now the pain is completely alleviated." The pain did not return.

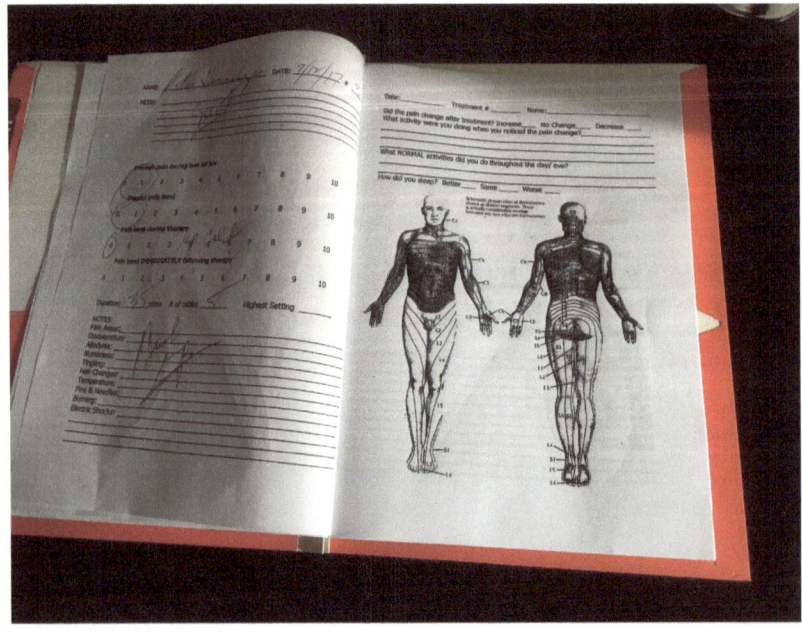

RUTHERFORD ALLIED MEDICAL GROUP

323 Union Avenue, Rutherford, New Jersey

The Rutherford Allied Medical office is an unpretentious building located in the middle of town across the street from a Dunkin' Donuts and next to an Italian Pizza restaurant.

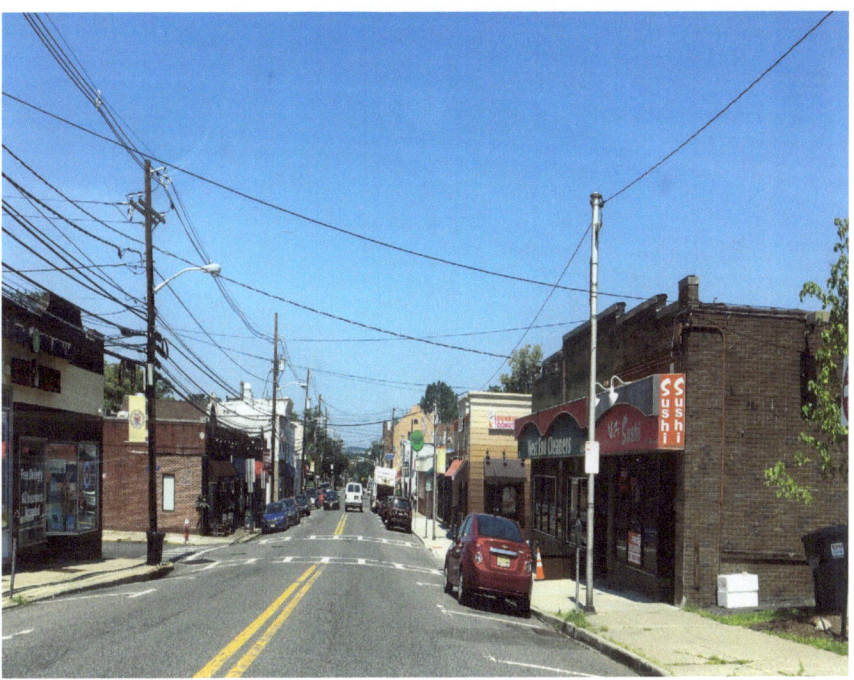

Yes, it is quite amazing that one man, Dr. Cooney, a small machine called Calmare® placed in a tiny treatment room in this little town in New Jersey could be so effective in treating RSD.

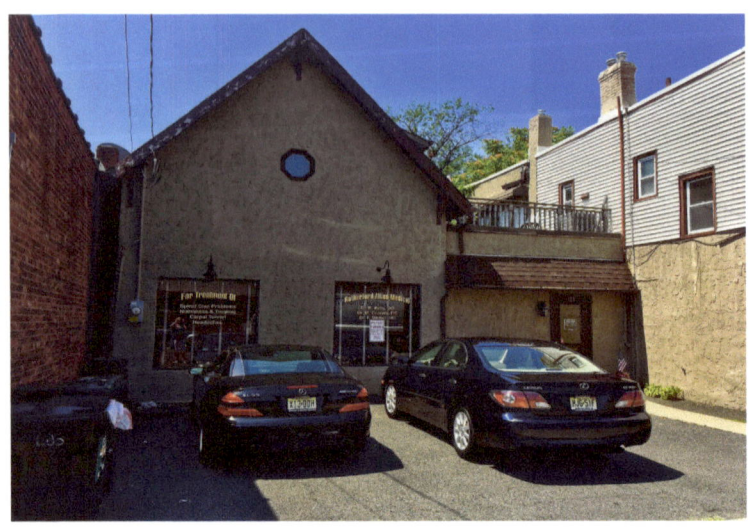

Dr. Cooney is a Remarkable Doctor!

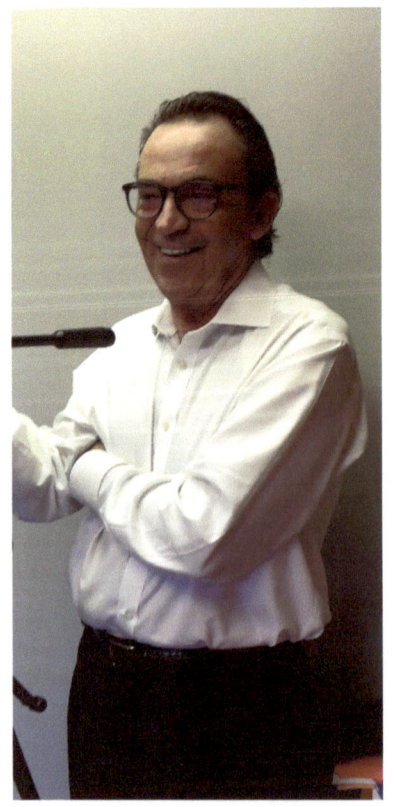

Dr. Cooney is upbeat and has a wealth of funny stories. He continues to learn and perfect the fine art of Calmare® Treatment through his questions and the attention he gives to each patient. I feel this attention to detail is what gives him the edge in his effective use of the Calmare® machine and treatment methods. His caring nature shows in his every action and word. The positioning of the electrodes is a very important component of the process. He personally administers each treatment because he believes that consistency is key to the success of the treatment.

Barbara and Cathy always greet us with a smile. They love working here. Cathy said, "I relish the miracles of joy I witness at this office each week with Dr. Cooney.

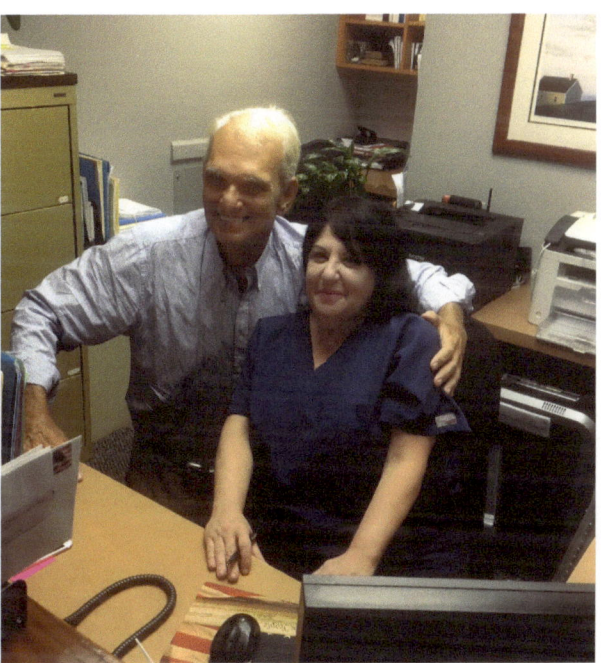

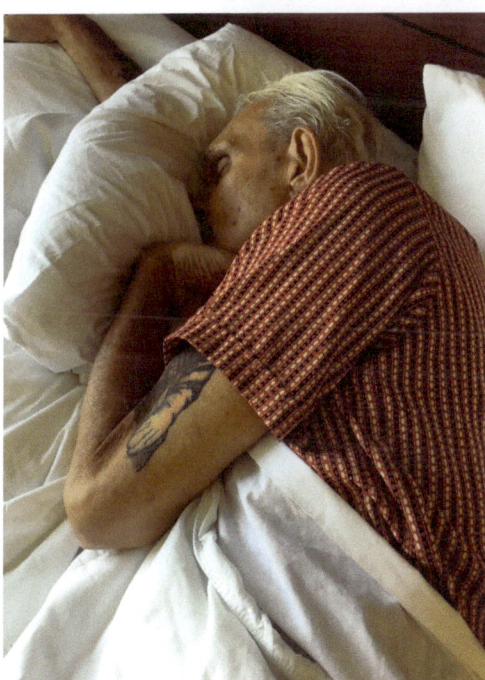

After treatments:

Sleep,

Sleep

and more

sleep!

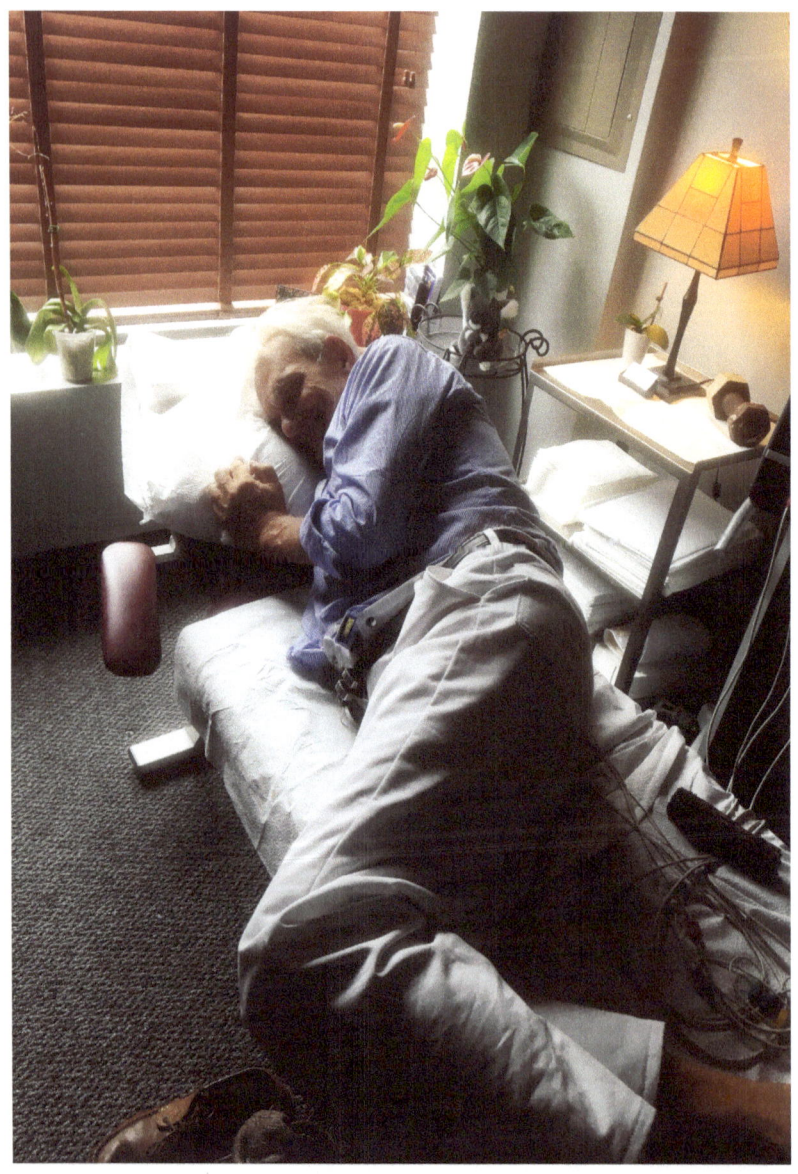

The second week of Calmare® Treatments continue in the same manner as the first week. The electrodes are positioned on Peter's foot and back in the same locations. The intensity of the electrodes are adjusted.

WEEK TWO

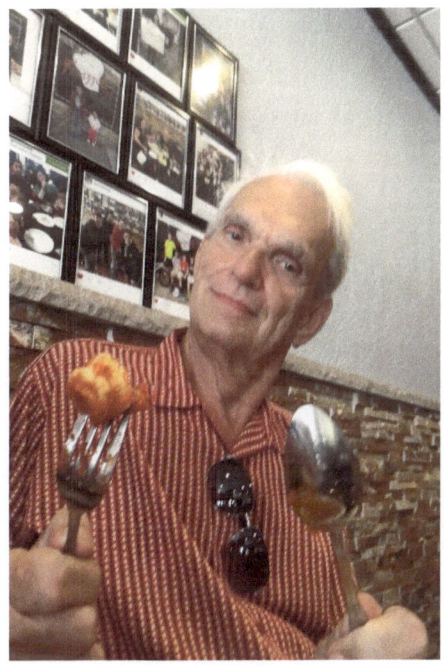

Peter's appetite is improving. Hungry and feeling "normal". Peter is learning to live life without a burning painful foot. Walking feels different. He can sit in a chair and be comfortable. The need to cringe and wince are gone.

The following are the Week 2 Daily Messages sent to family.

Monday, Week 2, Treatment 6:

All good! Peter is pain free. Peter is still very tired and sleepy. Dr. Cooney said that will stop when the treatments cease and he will most likely remain pain free or at a very low 1 or 2 level. If the pain returns in the future a booster treatment will take care if it. Pain Free! This opens so many doors and avenues of possibilities for Peter and I! 😊

Tuesday, Week 2, Treatment 7:

There was a return of the burning sensation last night around 1:00AM (level 5) A pain pill was taken. This morning a mild burning continued. We had the complimentary breakfast this morning. Peter felt awake and comfortable enough to go out to lunch prior to treatment. This is the first time we have been out of the hotel other than for treatments. Hungry. Peter cleared his plate of salad, steak, fries, and a spinach side dish. He is consuming a lot of food.

Treatment today was the usual with the addition of rolling the bottom of the foot on a tube cushion to further stimulate the non pain nerve sensors. Peter left the office pain free. Now we are back at the hotel and he is asleep.

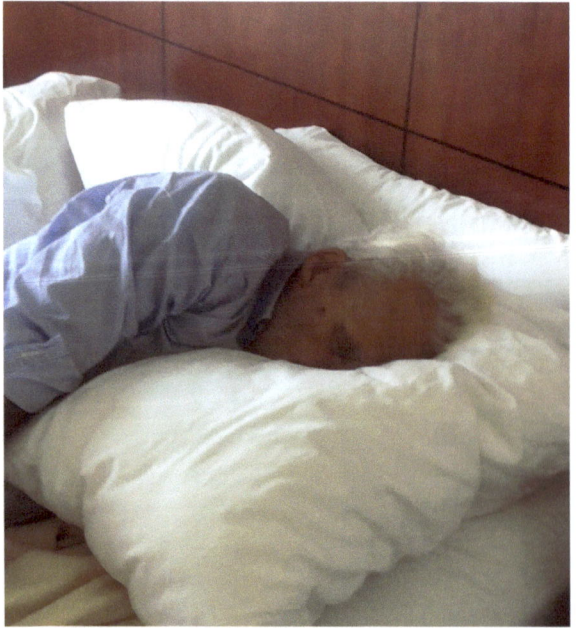

Wednesday, Week 2, Treatment 8:

Peter is feeling NORMAL. The pain and burning are nonexistent and Dr. Cooney is surprised, saying it is "extraordinary at this stage". The persistent feeling of numbness is, as of today, gone. Sleepiness continues but I notice he is awake more hours, alert, and his energy has increased.

Peter is beyond happy!

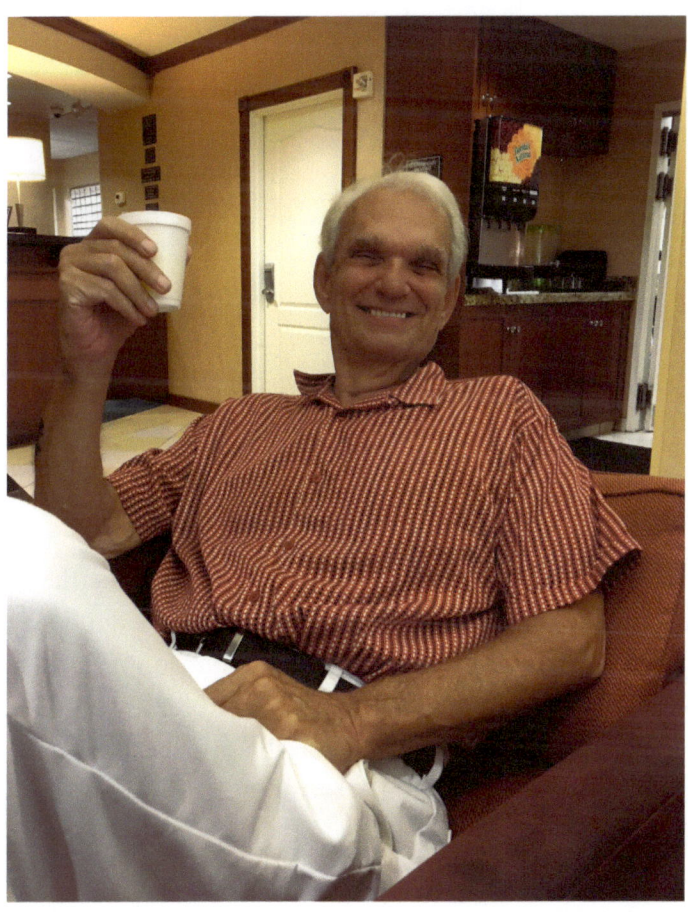

Thursday, Week 2, Treatment 9:

The extreme need for sleep continues. Dr. Cooney keeps on stressing that sleeping is an important part of the healing process. "Don't push yourself!" he says to Peter in his firm Doctor Voice. The pattern for the past few days is: Peter is awake a bit in the morning after breakfast, then back to sleep around 10. Awake again around noon for an hour or 2 (for treatment and lunch) then sleeps the entire afternoon till around 5-6. I wake him for dinner. He is out for the night, around 8.

When he is awake he is feeling really good and pain free, but has little energy and feels fuzzy in his thinking.

He is eating well. He has not taken a pain pill for 2 days. As a result, there are some side effects.

Friday, Week 2, Treatment 10:

Peter mentioned to the Dr. Cooney that he felt ready to go back to the gym. The Doctor, in an a typical stern voice, told Peter to take it easy for the next 10-14 days. No pain does not mean your foot is healed.

Dr. Cooney referenced getting hit in the eye. It hurts, the hurt goes away but just look in the mirror at that black eye and you know it is not healed. "Be very careful with your foot Peter!" he said. "An injury could entice the burning pain to return. If it does return to a level 3 in the future come into the office immediately for two to four booster treatments."

Feeling no pain for hours, then days, then weeks, then months is something that had not occurred in 17 years of searching. Life is a treasure and being pain free is a gift that inspires us to appreciate every moment of each day, each other, our children and grandchildren, the people we enjoy and our surroundings.

It is a happy adjustment as we look forward to life without the burning intense pain Peter endured for so long. We do not know how long this freedom from pain will last. A degree of pain could return. Booster treatments alleviate some of the fear.

Peter has an occasional slight return of discomfort in his right foot. A pain pill removes the pain within a half hour. The pain remains completely abated for days.

Seven weeks after the 10th Calmare® treatment the RSD monster reared his evil head. Peter woke in the middle of the night with a burning 7-8 pain in his right foot. Fear and depression griped him. Dr. Cooney had stated to let him know immediately if the pain reoccurs. After a call to Dr. Cooney and two booster treatments Peter is blissfully pain free again.

With love and a renewed zest for living,

Judy + Peter

Life is Good!

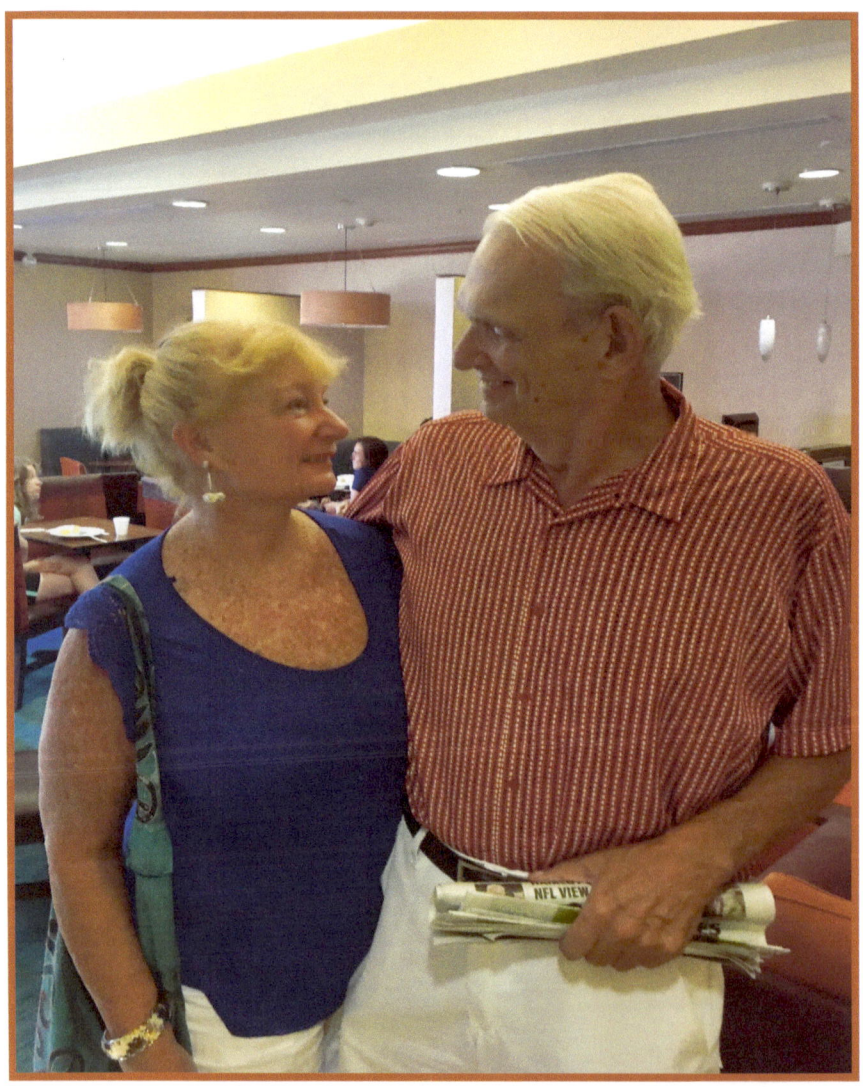

You can contact us at this email address that we have designated for questions regarding this book.

PeterRSDCalmare@aol.com